Simply Me

A Daily Food Journal for the 17 Day Diet &
Other Fun Prompts to Help You Stay on Track

Torey Lynn
Creator of Simply17™

DEDICATION

Losing weight is a life long journey for most of us. This journal was created for the person who needs a bit of a helping hand. The Simply Me journal is dedicated to you!

CONTENTS

ACKNOWLEDGMENTS

I want to acknowledge all of the ladies (and a few gentlemen, too!) who are a part of my blog community. Some have been on this ride since the beginning (2011) and I appreciate every single one of you! You're the reason I keep doing what I do.

The only person you are destined to become is the person you decide to be.

- Ralph Waldo Emerson

Hello!

Introduction to Simply Me

Simply Me is a daily journal broken down into three cycles of 17 days each. Each cycle is broken into two parts: days one through eight and days nine through 17.

Each day you'll keep track of food and fluid intake, fitness activity, and other daily prompts such as affirmations, daily gratitude, and daily stats if you choose to measure and weigh daily.

At the beginning of each eight and nine day period, you'll find a "beginning stats" worksheet where you'll record your weight and inches and choose three mini goals you want to achieve for that specific time period.

At the end of each eight and nine day period, you'll find an "ending stats" worksheet where you'll record your weight and inches progress as well as celebrate your three wins from that specific time period.

At the end of each cycle (day 17), you'll find a worksheet to "reflect and review" your progress over the 17 day period.

There will be several areas within the journal to record your thoughts, desires, and feelings. There's even room to doodle if that's your thing! At the end of each cycle, you'll also have the opportunity to complete your gratitude journal.

Please have fun with your journal and enjoy your journey!

If you want additional resources such as meal plans and recipes, or a private community for extra support, make sure you check out my blog over here: 17ddblog.com

xoxo, Torey Lynn

Cycle 1

Days 1 – 8

I am open, ready and willing to receive the benefits of self discovery through a healthy lifestyle (including enjoying a lot fun experiences along the way!).

Beginning Stats

Cycle 1, Days 1 - 8

Date: _____

Weight: _____

Inches:

Neck: _____   Midriff: _____

Chest: _____   Hips: _____

Left Arm: _____   Left Thigh: _____

Mini Goals

I want to achieve the following 3 "mini goals" in the next 8 days:

1. _____

2. _____

3. _____

Random Thoughts, Ideas & Musings (drawings allowed, too!)

Working from the Inside Out

Cycle 1, Day 1 Date: _____

My Daily Intention: how do I want to feel today?

I Believe....I'll Repeat These 3 Affirmations Today:

1. _____

2. _____

3. _____

My Gratitude Journal (every day I list something new):

1. _____

2. _____

3. _____

My Daily Stats (optional):

Weight: _____   Blood Sugar: _____   Other: _____

Blood
Pressure: _____   Cholesterol: _____   Other: _____

My Daily Fitness Activity:

Activity	Duration

Daily Food Checklist & Journal

Cycle 1, Day 1 Date: _____	Daily Food Journal (Food Types and Quantities)
Breakfast: ☐ Protein and/or Probiotics ☐ Fruit	
Lunch: ☐ Protein and/or Probiotics ☐ Cleansing Vegetables	
Dinner: ☐ Protein ☐ Cleansing Vegetables	
Snacks: ☐ 2nd Probiotic ☐ 2nd Fruit before 2pm	
Friendly Fats (2 Servings): ☐ Olive/Flax Oil	

Daily Hydration Check	
Hot Lemon Water	☐
Plain Water	☐ ☐ ☐ ☐ ☐ ☐ ☐ ☐
Green Tea	☐ ☐ ☐

Working from the Inside Out

Cycle 1, Day 2 Date: _____

My Daily Intention: how do I want to feel today?

I Believe....I'll Repeat These 3 Affirmations Today:

1. _____

2. _____

3. _____

My Gratitude Journal (every day I list something new):

1. _____

2. _____

3. _____

My Daily Stats (optional):

Weight: _____   Blood Sugar: _____   Other: _____

Blood
Pressure: _____   Cholesterol: _____   Other: _____

My Daily Fitness Activity:

Activity	Duration

Daily Food Checklist & Journal

Cycle 1, Day 2 Date: _____	Daily Food Journal (Food Types and Quantities)
Breakfast: ☐ Protein and/or Probiotics ☐ Fruit	
Lunch: ☐ Protein and/or Probiotics ☐ Cleansing Vegetables	
Dinner: ☐ Protein ☐ Cleansing Vegetables	
Snacks: ☐ 2nd Probiotic ☐ 2nd Fruit before 2pm	
Friendly Fats (2 Servings): ☐ Olive/Flax Oil	

Daily Hydration Check	
Hot Lemon Water	☐
Plain Water	☐ ☐ ☐ ☐ ☐ ☐ ☐
Green Tea	☐ ☐ ☐

Working from the Inside Out

Cycle 1, Day 3 Date: _____

My Daily Intention: how do I want to feel today?

I Believe....I'll Repeat These 3 Affirmations Today:

1. _____

2. _____

3. _____

My Gratitude Journal (every day I list something new):

1. _____

2. _____

3. _____

My Daily Stats (optional):

Weight: _____   Blood Sugar: _____   Other: _____

Blood
Pressure: _____   Cholesterol: _____   Other: _____

My Daily Fitness Activity:

Activity	Duration

Daily Food Checklist & Journal

Cycle 1, Day 3 Date: _____	Daily Food Journal (Food Types and Quantities)
Breakfast: ☐ Protein and/or Probiotics ☐ Fruit	
Lunch: ☐ Protein and/or Probiotics ☐ Cleansing Vegetables	
Dinner: ☐ Protein ☐ Cleansing Vegetables	
Snacks: ☐ 2nd Probiotic ☐ 2nd Fruit before 2pm	
Friendly Fats (2 Servings): ☐ Olive/Flax Oil	

Daily Hydration Check	
Hot Lemon Water	☐
Plain Water	☐ ☐ ☐ ☐ ☐ ☐ ☐ ☐
Green Tea	☐ ☐ ☐

Working from the Inside Out

Cycle 1, Day 4 Date: _____

My Daily Intention: how do I want to feel today?

I Believe....I'll Repeat These 3 Affirmations Today:

1. _____

2. _____

3. _____

My Gratitude Journal (every day I list something new):

1. _____

2. _____

3. _____

My Daily Stats (optional):

Weight: _____   Blood Sugar: _____   Other: _____

Blood
Pressure: _____   Cholesterol: _____   Other: _____

My Daily Fitness Activity:

Activity	Duration

Daily Food Checklist & Journal

Cycle 1, Day 4 Date: _____	Daily Food Journal (Food Types and Quantities)
Breakfast: ☐ Protein and/or Probiotics ☐ Fruit	
Lunch: ☐ Protein and/or Probiotics ☐ Cleansing Vegetables	
Dinner: ☐ Protein ☐ Cleansing Vegetables	
Snacks: ☐ 2nd Probiotic ☐ 2nd Fruit before 2pm	
Friendly Fats (2 Servings): ☐ Olive/Flax Oil	

Daily Hydration Check	
Hot Lemon Water	☐
Plain Water	☐ ☐ ☐ ☐ ☐ ☐ ☐ ☐
Green Tea	☐ ☐ ☐

Working from the Inside Out

Cycle 1, Day 5 Date: _____

My Daily Intention: how do I want to feel today?

I Believe....I'll Repeat These 3 Affirmations Today:

1. _____

2. _____

3. _____

My Gratitude Journal (every day I list something new):

1. _____

2. _____

3. _____

My Daily Stats (optional):

Weight: _____   Blood Sugar: _____   Other: _____

Blood
Pressure: _____   Cholesterol: _____   Other: _____

My Daily Fitness Activity:

Activity	Duration

Daily Food Checklist & Journal

Cycle 1, Day 5 Date: _____	Daily Food Journal (Food Types and Quantities)
Breakfast: ☐ Protein and/or Probiotics ☐ Fruit	
Lunch: ☐ Protein and/or Probiotics ☐ Cleansing Vegetables	
Dinner: ☐ Protein ☐ Cleansing Vegetables	
Snacks: ☐ 2nd Probiotic ☐ 2nd Fruit before 2pm	
Friendly Fats (2 Servings): ☐ Olive/Flax Oil	

Daily Hydration Check	
Hot Lemon Water	☐
Plain Water	☐ ☐ ☐ ☐ ☐ ☐ ☐
Green Tea	☐ ☐ ☐

Working from the Inside Out

Cycle 1, Day 6 Date: _____

My Daily Intention: how do I want to feel today?

I Believe....I'll Repeat These 3 Affirmations Today:

1. _____

2. _____

3. _____

My Gratitude Journal (every day I list something new):

1. _____

2. _____

3. _____

My Daily Stats (optional):

Weight: _____   Blood Sugar: _____   Other: _____

Blood
Pressure: _____   Cholesterol: _____   Other: _____

My Daily Fitness Activity:

Activity	Duration

Daily Food Checklist & Journal

Cycle 1, Day 6 Date: _____	Daily Food Journal (Food Types and Quantities)
Breakfast: ☐ Protein and/or Probiotics ☐ Fruit	
Lunch: ☐ Protein and/or Probiotics ☐ Cleansing Vegetables	
Dinner: ☐ Protein ☐ Cleansing Vegetables	
Snacks: ☐ 2nd Probiotic ☐ 2nd Fruit before 2pm	
Friendly Fats (2 Servings): ☐ Olive/Flax Oil	

Daily Hydration Check	
Hot Lemon Water	☐
Plain Water	☐ ☐ ☐ ☐ ☐ ☐ ☐
Green Tea	☐ ☐ ☐

Working from the Inside Out

Cycle 1, Day 7 Date: _____

My Daily Intention: how do I want to feel today?

I Believe....I'll Repeat These 3 Affirmations Today:

1. _____

2. _____

3. _____

My Gratitude Journal (every day I list something new):

1. _____

2. _____

3. _____

My Daily Stats (optional):

Weight: _____   Blood Sugar: _____   Other: _____

Blood
Pressure: _____   Cholesterol: _____   Other: _____

My Daily Fitness Activity:

Activity	Duration

Daily Food Checklist & Journal

Cycle 1, Day 7 Date: _____	Daily Food Journal (Food Types and Quantities)
Breakfast: ☐ Protein and/or Probiotics ☐ Fruit	
Lunch: ☐ Protein and/or Probiotics ☐ Cleansing Vegetables	
Dinner: ☐ Protein ☐ Cleansing Vegetables	
Snacks: ☐ 2nd Probiotic ☐ 2nd Fruit before 2pm	
Friendly Fats (2 Servings): ☐ Olive/Flax Oil	

Daily Hydration Check	
Hot Lemon Water	☐
Plain Water	☐ ☐ ☐ ☐ ☐ ☐ ☐ ☐
Green Tea	☐ ☐ ☐

Working from the Inside Out

Cycle 1, Day 8 Date: _____

My Daily Intention: how do I want to feel today?

I Believe....I'll Repeat These 3 Affirmations Today:

1. _____

2. _____

3. _____

My Gratitude Journal (every day I list something new):

1. _____

2. _____

3. _____

My Daily Stats (optional):

Weight: _____   Blood Sugar: _____   Other: _____

Blood
Pressure: _____   Cholesterol: _____   Other: _____

My Daily Fitness Activity:

Activity	Duration

Daily Food Checklist & Journal

Cycle 1, Day 8 Date: _____	Daily Food Journal (Food Types and Quantities)
Breakfast: ☐ Protein and/or Probiotics ☐ Fruit	
Lunch: ☐ Protein and/or Probiotics ☐ Cleansing Vegetables	
Dinner: ☐ Protein ☐ Cleansing Vegetables	
Snacks: ☐ 2nd Probiotic ☐ 2nd Fruit before 2pm	
Friendly Fats (2 Servings): ☐ Olive/Flax Oil	

Daily Hydration Check	
Hot Lemon Water	☐
Plain Water	☐ ☐ ☐ ☐ ☐ ☐ ☐
Green Tea	☐ ☐ ☐

Ending Stats
Cycle 1, Days 1 - 8

Date: _____

Weight: _____

Inches:

Neck: _____   Midriff: _____

Chest: _____   Hips: _____

Left Arm: _____   Left Thigh: _____

My Wins

I celebrate the following wins (both big and small) from the last 8 days:

1. _____

2. _____

3. _____

Random Thoughts, Ideas & Musings (drawings allowed, too!)

Cycle 1

Days 9 – 17

I am motivated by the physical changes I see in my body (and mind) and I am open to continuing to living a life in a healthy and enjoyable way.

Beginning Stats

Cycle 1, Days 9 - 17

Date: _____

Weight: _____

Inches:

Neck: _____   Midriff: _____

Chest: _____   Hips: _____

Left Arm: _____   Left Thigh: _____

Mini Goals

I want to achieve the following 3 "mini goals" in the next 9 days:

1. _____

2. _____

3. _____

Random Thoughts, Ideas & Musings (drawings allowed, too!)

Working from the Inside Out

Cycle 1, Day 9 Date: _____

My Daily Intention: how do I want to feel today?

I Believe....I'll Repeat These 3 Affirmations Today:

1. _____

2. _____

3. _____

My Gratitude Journal (every day I list something new):

1. _____

2. _____

3. _____

My Daily Stats (optional):

Weight: _____ Blood Sugar: _____ Other: _____

Blood
Pressure: _____ Cholesterol: _____ Other: _____

My Daily Fitness Activity:

Activity	Duration

Daily Food Checklist & Journal

Cycle 1, Day 9 Date: _____	Daily Food Journal (Food Types and Quantities)
Breakfast: ☐ Protein and/or Probiotics ☐ Fruit	
Lunch: ☐ Protein and/or Probiotics ☐ Cleansing Vegetables	
Dinner: ☐ Protein ☐ Cleansing Vegetables	
Snacks: ☐ 2nd Probiotic ☐ 2nd Fruit before 2pm	
Friendly Fats (2 Servings): ☐ Olive/Flax Oil	

Daily Hydration Check	
Hot Lemon Water	☐
Plain Water	☐ ☐ ☐ ☐ ☐ ☐ ☐
Green Tea	☐ ☐ ☐

Working from the Inside Out

Cycle 1, Day 10 Date: _____

My Daily Intention: how do I want to feel today?

I Believe....I'll Repeat These 3 Affirmations Today:

1. _____

2. _____

3. _____

My Gratitude Journal (every day I list something new):

1. _____

2. _____

3. _____

My Daily Stats (optional):

Weight: _____   Blood Sugar: _____   Other: _____

Blood
Pressure: _____   Cholesterol: _____   Other: _____

My Daily Fitness Activity:

Activity	Duration

Daily Food Checklist & Journal

Cycle 1, Day 10 Date: _____	Daily Food Journal (Food Types and Quantities)
Breakfast: ☐ Protein and/or Probiotics ☐ Fruit	
Lunch: ☐ Protein and/or Probiotics ☐ Cleansing Vegetables	
Dinner: ☐ Protein ☐ Cleansing Vegetables	
Snacks: ☐ 2nd Probiotic ☐ 2nd Fruit before 2pm	
Friendly Fats (2 Servings): ☐ Olive/Flax Oil	

Daily Hydration Check	
Hot Lemon Water	☐
Plain Water	☐ ☐ ☐ ☐ ☐ ☐ ☐
Green Tea	☐ ☐ ☐

Working from the Inside Out

Cycle 1, Day 11 Date: _____

My Daily Intention: how do I want to feel today?

I Believe....I'll Repeat These 3 Affirmations Today:

1. _____

2. _____

3. _____

My Gratitude Journal (every day I list something new):

1. _____

2. _____

3. _____

My Daily Stats (optional):

Weight: _____   Blood Sugar: _____   Other: _____

Blood
Pressure: _____   Cholesterol: _____   Other: _____

My Daily Fitness Activity:

Activity	Duration

Daily Food Checklist & Journal

Cycle 1, Day 11 Date: _____	Daily Food Journal (Food Types and Quantities)
Breakfast: ☐ Protein and/or Probiotics ☐ Fruit	
Lunch: ☐ Protein and/or Probiotics ☐ Cleansing Vegetables	
Dinner: ☐ Protein ☐ Cleansing Vegetables	
Snacks: ☐ 2nd Probiotic ☐ 2nd Fruit before 2pm	
Friendly Fats (2 Servings): ☐ Olive/Flax Oil	

Daily Hydration Check	
Hot Lemon Water	☐
Plain Water	☐ ☐ ☐ ☐ ☐ ☐ ☐ ☐
Green Tea	☐ ☐ ☐

Working from the Inside Out

Cycle 1, Day 12 Date: _____

My Daily Intention: how do I want to feel today?

I Believe....I'll Repeat These 3 Affirmations Today:

1. _____

2. _____

3. _____

My Gratitude Journal (every day I list something new):

1. _____

2. _____

3. _____

My Daily Stats (optional):

Weight: _____   Blood Sugar: _____   Other: _____

Blood
Pressure: _____   Cholesterol: _____   Other: _____

My Daily Fitness Activity:

Activity	Duration

Daily Food Checklist & Journal

Cycle 1, Day 12 Date: _____	Daily Food Journal (Food Types and Quantities)
Breakfast: ☐ Protein and/or Probiotics ☐ Fruit	
Lunch: ☐ Protein and/or Probiotics ☐ Cleansing Vegetables	
Dinner: ☐ Protein ☐ Cleansing Vegetables	
Snacks: ☐ 2nd Probiotic ☐ 2nd Fruit before 2pm	
Friendly Fats (2 Servings): ☐ Olive/Flax Oil	

Daily Hydration Check	
Hot Lemon Water	☐
Plain Water	☐ ☐ ☐ ☐ ☐ ☐ ☐ ☐
Green Tea	☐ ☐ ☐

Working from the Inside Out

Cycle 1, Day 13 Date: _____

My Daily Intention: how do I want to feel today?

I Believe....I'll Repeat These 3 Affirmations Today:

1. _____

2. _____

3. _____

My Gratitude Journal (every day I list something new):

1. _____

2. _____

3. _____

My Daily Stats (optional):

Weight: _____   Blood Sugar: _____   Other: _____

Blood
Pressure: _____   Cholesterol: _____   Other: _____

My Daily Fitness Activity:

Activity	Duration

Daily Food Checklist & Journal

Cycle 1, Day 13 Date: _____	Daily Food Journal (Food Types and Quantities)
Breakfast: ☐ Protein and/or Probiotics ☐ Fruit	
Lunch: ☐ Protein and/or Probiotics ☐ Cleansing Vegetables	
Dinner: ☐ Protein ☐ Cleansing Vegetables	
Snacks: ☐ 2nd Probiotic ☐ 2nd Fruit before 2pm	
Friendly Fats (2 Servings): ☐ Olive/Flax Oil	

Daily Hydration Check	
Hot Lemon Water	☐
Plain Water	☐ ☐ ☐ ☐ ☐ ☐ ☐
Green Tea	☐ ☐ ☐

Working from the Inside Out

Cycle 1, Day 14 Date: _____

My Daily Intention: how do I want to feel today?

I Believe....I'll Repeat These 3 Affirmations Today:

1. _____

2. _____

3. _____

My Gratitude Journal (every day I list something new):

1. _____

2. _____

3. _____

My Daily Stats (optional):

Weight: _____   Blood Sugar: _____   Other: _____

Blood
Pressure: _____   Cholesterol: _____   Other: _____

My Daily Fitness Activity:

Activity	Duration

Daily Food Checklist & Journal

Cycle 1, Day 14 Date: _____	Daily Food Journal (Food Types and Quantities)
Breakfast: ☐ Protein and/or Probiotics ☐ Fruit	
Lunch: ☐ Protein and/or Probiotics ☐ Cleansing Vegetables	
Dinner: ☐ Protein ☐ Cleansing Vegetables	
Snacks: ☐ 2nd Probiotic ☐ 2nd Fruit before 2pm	
Friendly Fats (2 Servings): ☐ Olive/Flax Oil	

Daily Hydration Check	
Hot Lemon Water	☐
Plain Water	☐ ☐ ☐ ☐ ☐ ☐ ☐
Green Tea	☐ ☐ ☐

Working from the Inside Out

Cycle 1, Day 15 Date: _____

My Daily Intention: how do I want to feel today?

I Believe....I'll Repeat These 3 Affirmations Today:

1. _____

2. _____

3. _____

My Gratitude Journal (every day I list something new):

1. _____

2. _____

3. _____

My Daily Stats (optional):

Weight: _____   Blood Sugar: _____   Other: _____

Blood
Pressure: _____   Cholesterol: _____   Other: _____

My Daily Fitness Activity:

Activity	Duration

Daily Food Checklist & Journal

Cycle 1, Day 15 Date: _____	Daily Food Journal (Food Types and Quantities)
Breakfast: ☐ Protein and/or Probiotics ☐ Fruit	
Lunch: ☐ Protein and/or Probiotics ☐ Cleansing Vegetables	
Dinner: ☐ Protein ☐ Cleansing Vegetables	
Snacks: ☐ 2nd Probiotic ☐ 2nd Fruit before 2pm	
Friendly Fats (2 Servings): ☐ Olive/Flax Oil	

Daily Hydration Check	
Hot Lemon Water	☐
Plain Water	☐ ☐ ☐ ☐ ☐ ☐ ☐
Green Tea	☐ ☐ ☐

Working from the Inside Out

Cycle 1, Day 16 Date: _____

My Daily Intention: how do I want to feel today?

I Believe....I'll Repeat These 3 Affirmations Today:

1. _____

2. _____

3. _____

My Gratitude Journal (every day I list something new):

1. _____

2. _____

3. _____

My Daily Stats (optional):

Weight: _____   Blood Sugar: _____   Other: _____

Blood
Pressure: _____   Cholesterol: _____   Other: _____

My Daily Fitness Activity:

Activity	Duration

Daily Food Checklist & Journal

Cycle 1, Day 16 Date: _____	Daily Food Journal (Food Types and Quantities)
Breakfast: ☐ Protein and/or Probiotics ☐ Fruit	
Lunch: ☐ Protein and/or Probiotics ☐ Cleansing Vegetables	
Dinner: ☐ Protein ☐ Cleansing Vegetables	
Snacks: ☐ 2nd Probiotic ☐ 2nd Fruit before 2pm	
Friendly Fats (2 Servings): ☐ Olive/Flax Oil	

Daily Hydration Check	
Hot Lemon Water	☐
Plain Water	☐ ☐ ☐ ☐ ☐ ☐ ☐
Green Tea	☐ ☐ ☐

Working from the Inside Out

Cycle 1, Day 17 Date: _____

My Daily Intention: how do I want to feel today?

I Believe....I'll Repeat These 3 Affirmations Today:

1. _____

2. _____

3. _____

My Gratitude Journal (every day I list something new):

1. _____

2. _____

3. _____

My Daily Stats (optional):

Weight: _____   Blood Sugar: _____   Other: _____

Blood
Pressure: _____   Cholesterol: _____   Other: _____

My Daily Fitness Activity:

Activity	Duration

Daily Food Checklist & Journal

Cycle 1, Day 17 Date: _____	Daily Food Journal (Food Types and Quantities)
Breakfast: ☐ Protein and/or Probiotics ☐ Fruit	
Lunch: ☐ Protein and/or Probiotics ☐ Cleansing Vegetables	
Dinner: ☐ Protein ☐ Cleansing Vegetables	
Snacks: ☐ 2nd Probiotic ☐ 2nd Fruit before 2pm	
Friendly Fats (2 Servings): ☐ Olive/Flax Oil	

Daily Hydration Check	
Hot Lemon Water	☐
Plain Water	☐ ☐ ☐ ☐ ☐ ☐ ☐ ☐
Green Tea	☐ ☐ ☐

Ending Stats
Cycle 1, Days 9 - 17

Date: _____

Weight: _____

Inches:

Neck: _____   Midriff: _____

Chest: _____   Hips: _____

Left Arm: _____   Left Thigh: _____

My Wins

I celebrate the following wins (both big and small) from the last 9 days:

1. _____

2. _____

3. _____

Random Thoughts, Ideas & Musings (drawings allowed, too!)

Reflect & Review
Cycle 1, Days 1 – 17

	Beginning Stats	**Ending Stats**	**Difference**
Weight			
Inches:			
Neck			
Chest			
Left Arm			
Midriff			
Hips			
Left Thigh			

The 1 Thing

During the last 17 days of this cycle, I learned the following about myself...

Gratitude Journal

Cycle 2

Days 1 – 8

I am fully aware and accept that the scale does not tell my whole story. My body is changing, even if the number on the scale does not necessarily reflect my progress. I'm sleeping better, I have more energy and my mind is clear. I'm building the foundation of a healthy way of living.

Beginning Stats

Cycle 2, Days 1 - 8

Date: _____

Weight: _____

Inches:

Neck: _____   Midriff: _____

Chest: _____   Hips: _____

Left Arm: _____   Left Thigh: _____

Mini Goals

I want to achieve the following 3 "mini goals" in the next 8 days:

1. _____

2. _____

3. _____

Random Thoughts, Ideas & Musings (drawings allowed, too!)

Working from the Inside Out

Cycle 2, Day 1 Date: _____

My Daily Intention: how do I want to feel today?

I Believe....I'll Repeat These 3 Affirmations Today:

1. _____

2. _____

3. _____

My Gratitude Journal (every day I list something new):

1. _____

2. _____

3. _____

My Daily Stats (optional):

Weight: _____   Blood Sugar: _____   Other: _____

Blood
Pressure: _____   Cholesterol: _____   Other: _____

My Daily Fitness Activity:

Activity	Duration

Daily Food Checklist & Journal

Cycle 2, Day 1 Date: _____ (Activate Day)	Daily Food Journal (Food Types and Quantities)
Breakfast: ☐ Protein and/or Probiotics ☐ Fruit ☐ Natural Starch	
Lunch: ☐ Protein and/or Probiotics ☐ Cleansing Vegetables ☐ Natural Starch	
Dinner: ☐ Protein ☐ Cleansing Vegetables	
Snacks: ☐ 2nd Probiotic ☐ 2nd Fruit before 2pm	
Friendly Fats (2 Servings): ☐ Olive/Flax Oil	

Daily Hydration Check	
Hot Lemon Water	☐
Plain Water	☐ ☐ ☐ ☐ ☐ ☐ ☐ ☐
Green Tea	☐ ☐ ☐

Working from the Inside Out

Cycle 2, Day 2 Date: _____

My Daily Intention: how do I want to feel today?

I Believe....I'll Repeat These 3 Affirmations Today:

1. _____

2. _____

3. _____

My Gratitude Journal (every day I list something new):

1. _____

2. _____

3. _____

My Daily Stats (optional):

Weight: _____ Blood Sugar: _____ Other: _____

Blood
Pressure: _____ Cholesterol: _____ Other: _____

My Daily Fitness Activity:

Activity	Duration

Daily Food Checklist & Journal

Cycle 2, Day 2 Date: _____ (Accelerate Day)	Daily Food Journal (Food Types and Quantities)
Breakfast: ☐ Protein and/or Probiotics ☐ Fruit	
Lunch: ☐ Protein and/or Probiotics ☐ Cleansing Vegetables	
Dinner: ☐ Protein ☐ Cleansing Vegetables	
Snacks: ☐ 2nd Probiotic ☐ 2nd Fruit before 2pm	
Friendly Fats (2 Servings): ☐ Olive/Flax Oil	

Daily Hydration Check	
Hot Lemon Water	☐
Plain Water	☐ ☐ ☐ ☐ ☐ ☐ ☐
Green Tea	☐ ☐ ☐

Working from the Inside Out

Cycle 2, Day 3 Date: _____

My Daily Intention: how do I want to feel today?

I Believe....I'll Repeat These 3 Affirmations Today:

1. _____

2. _____

3. _____

My Gratitude Journal (every day I list something new):

1. _____

2. _____

3. _____

My Daily Stats (optional):

Weight: _____   Blood Sugar: _____   Other: _____

Blood
Pressure: _____   Cholesterol: _____   Other: _____

My Daily Fitness Activity:

Activity	Duration

Daily Food Checklist & Journal

Cycle 2, Day 3 Date: _____ (Activate Day)	Daily Food Journal (Food Types and Quantities)
Breakfast: ☐ Protein and/or Probiotics ☐ Fruit ☐ Natural Starch	
Lunch: ☐ Protein and/or Probiotics ☐ Cleansing Vegetables ☐ Natural Starch	
Dinner: ☐ Protein ☐ Cleansing Vegetables	
Snacks: ☐ 2nd Probiotic ☐ 2nd Fruit before 2pm	
Friendly Fats (2 Servings): ☐ Olive/Flax Oil	

Daily Hydration Check	
Hot Lemon Water	☐
Plain Water	☐ ☐ ☐ ☐ ☐ ☐ ☐ ☐
Green Tea	☐ ☐ ☐

Working from the Inside Out

Cycle 2, Day 4 Date: _____

My Daily Intention: how do I want to feel today?

I Believe....I'll Repeat These 3 Affirmations Today:

1. _____

2. _____

3. _____

My Gratitude Journal (every day I list something new):

1. _____

2. _____

3. _____

My Daily Stats (optional):

Weight: _____   Blood Sugar: _____   Other: _____

Blood
Pressure: _____   Cholesterol: _____   Other: _____

My Daily Fitness Activity:

Activity	Duration

Daily Food Checklist & Journal

Cycle 2, Day 4 Date: _____ (Accelerate Day)	Daily Food Journal (Food Types and Quantities)
Breakfast: ☐ Protein and/or Probiotics ☐ Fruit	
Lunch: ☐ Protein and/or Probiotics ☐ Cleansing Vegetables	
Dinner: ☐ Protein ☐ Cleansing Vegetables	
Snacks: ☐ 2nd Probiotic ☐ 2nd Fruit before 2pm	
Friendly Fats (2 Servings): ☐ Olive/Flax Oil	

Daily Hydration Check	
Hot Lemon Water	☐
Plain Water	☐ ☐ ☐ ☐ ☐ ☐ ☐ ☐
Green Tea	☐ ☐ ☐

Working from the Inside Out

Cycle 2, Day 5 Date: _____

My Daily Intention: how do I want to feel today?

I Believe....I'll Repeat These 3 Affirmations Today:

1. _____

2. _____

3. _____

My Gratitude Journal (every day I list something new):

1. _____

2. _____

3. _____

My Daily Stats (optional):

Weight: _____   Blood Sugar: _____   Other: _____

Blood
Pressure: _____   Cholesterol: _____   Other: _____

My Daily Fitness Activity:

Activity	Duration

Daily Food Checklist & Journal

Cycle 2, Day 5 Date: _____ (Activate Day)	Daily Food Journal (Food Types and Quantities)
Breakfast: ☐ Protein and/or Probiotics ☐ Fruit ☐ Natural Starch	
Lunch: ☐ Protein and/or Probiotics ☐ Cleansing Vegetables ☐ Natural Starch	
Dinner: ☐ Protein ☐ Cleansing Vegetables	
Snacks: ☐ 2nd Probiotic ☐ 2nd Fruit before 2pm	
Friendly Fats (2 Servings): ☐ Olive/Flax Oil	

Daily Hydration Check	
Hot Lemon Water	☐
Plain Water	☐ ☐ ☐ ☐ ☐ ☐ ☐ ☐
Green Tea	☐ ☐ ☐

Working from the Inside Out

Cycle 2, Day 6 Date: _____

My Daily Intention: how do I want to feel today?

I Believe....I'll Repeat These 3 Affirmations Today:

1. _____

2. _____

3. _____

My Gratitude Journal (every day I list something new):

1. _____

2. _____

3. _____

My Daily Stats (optional):

Weight: _____   Blood Sugar: _____   Other: _____

Blood
Pressure: _____   Cholesterol: _____   Other: _____

My Daily Fitness Activity:

Activity	Duration

Daily Food Checklist & Journal

Cycle 2, Day 6 Date: _____ (Accelerate Day)	Daily Food Journal (Food Types and Quantities)
Breakfast: ☐ Protein and/or Probiotics ☐ Fruit	
Lunch: ☐ Protein and/or Probiotics ☐ Cleansing Vegetables	
Dinner: ☐ Protein ☐ Cleansing Vegetables	
Snacks: ☐ 2nd Probiotic ☐ 2nd Fruit before 2pm	
Friendly Fats (2 Servings): ☐ Olive/Flax Oil	

Daily Hydration Check	
Hot Lemon Water	☐
Plain Water	☐ ☐ ☐ ☐ ☐ ☐ ☐
Green Tea	☐ ☐ ☐

Working from the Inside Out

Cycle 2, Day 7 Date: _____

My Daily Intention: how do I want to feel today?

I Believe....I'll Repeat These 3 Affirmations Today:

1. _____

2. _____

3. _____

My Gratitude Journal (every day I list something new):

1. _____

2. _____

3. _____

My Daily Stats (optional):

Weight: _____   Blood Sugar: _____   Other: _____

Blood
Pressure: _____   Cholesterol: _____   Other: _____

My Daily Fitness Activity:

Activity	Duration

Daily Food Checklist & Journal

Cycle 2, Day 7 Date: _____ (Activate Day)	Daily Food Journal (Food Types and Quantities)
Breakfast: ☐ Protein and/or Probiotics ☐ Fruit ☐ Natural Starch	
Lunch: ☐ Protein and/or Probiotics ☐ Cleansing Vegetables ☐ Natural Starch	
Dinner: ☐ Protein ☐ Cleansing Vegetables	
Snacks: ☐ 2nd Probiotic ☐ 2nd Fruit before 2pm	
Friendly Fats (2 Servings): ☐ Olive/Flax Oil	

Daily Hydration Check	
Hot Lemon Water	☐
Plain Water	☐ ☐ ☐ ☐ ☐ ☐ ☐ ☐
Green Tea	☐ ☐ ☐

Working from the Inside Out

Cycle 2, Day 8 Date: _____

My Daily Intention: how do I want to feel today?

I Believe....I'll Repeat These 3 Affirmations Today:

1. _____

2. _____

3. _____

My Gratitude Journal (every day I list something new):

1. _____

2. _____

3. _____

My Daily Stats (optional):

Weight: _____   Blood Sugar: _____   Other: _____

Blood
Pressure: _____   Cholesterol: _____   Other: _____

My Daily Fitness Activity:

Activity	Duration

Daily Food Checklist & Journal

Cycle 2, Day 8 Date: _____ (Accelerate Day)	Daily Food Journal (Food Types and Quantities)
Breakfast: ☐ Protein and/or Probiotics ☐ Fruit	
Lunch: ☐ Protein and/or Probiotics ☐ Cleansing Vegetables	
Dinner: ☐ Protein ☐ Cleansing Vegetables	
Snacks: ☐ 2nd Probiotic ☐ 2nd Fruit before 2pm	
Friendly Fats (2 Servings): ☐ Olive/Flax Oil	

Daily Hydration Check	
Hot Lemon Water	☐
Plain Water	☐ ☐ ☐ ☐ ☐ ☐ ☐
Green Tea	☐ ☐ ☐

Ending Stats
Cycle 2, Days 1 - 8

Date: _____

Weight: _____

Inches:

Neck: _____   Midriff: _____

Chest: _____   Hips: _____

Left Arm: _____   Left Thigh: _____

My Wins

I celebrate the following wins (both big and small) from the last 8 days:

1. _____

2. _____

3. _____

Random Thoughts, Ideas & Musings (drawings allowed, too!)

Cycle 2

Days 9 – 17

I am becoming mentally, physically and emotionally stronger every day.

Beginning Stats

Cycle 2, Days 9 - 17

Date: _____

Weight: _____

Inches:

Neck: _____   Midriff: _____

Chest: _____   Hips: _____

Left Arm: _____   Left Thigh: _____

Mini Goals

I want to achieve the following 3 "mini goals" in the next 9 days:

1. _____

2. _____

3. _____

Random Thoughts, Ideas & Musings (drawings allowed, too!)

Working from the Inside Out

Cycle 2, Day 9 Date: _____

My Daily Intention: how do I want to feel today?

I Believe....I'll Repeat These 3 Affirmations Today:

1. _____

2. _____

3. _____

My Gratitude Journal (every day I list something new):

1. _____

2. _____

3. _____

My Daily Stats (optional):

Weight: _____   Blood Sugar: _____   Other: _____

Blood
Pressure: _____   Cholesterol: _____   Other: _____

My Daily Fitness Activity:

Activity	Duration

Daily Food Checklist & Journal

Cycle 2, Day 9 Date: _____ (Activate Day)	Daily Food Journal (Food Types and Quantities)
Breakfast: ☐ Protein and/or Probiotics ☐ Fruit ☐ Natural Starch	
Lunch: ☐ Protein and/or Probiotics ☐ Cleansing Vegetables ☐ Natural Starch	
Dinner: ☐ Protein ☐ Cleansing Vegetables	
Snacks: ☐ 2nd Probiotic ☐ 2nd Fruit before 2pm	
Friendly Fats (2 Servings): ☐ Olive/Flax Oil	

Daily Hydration Check	
Hot Lemon Water	☐
Plain Water	☐ ☐ ☐ ☐ ☐ ☐ ☐
Green Tea	☐ ☐ ☐

Working from the Inside Out

Cycle 2, Day 10 Date: _____

My Daily Intention: how do I want to feel today?

I Believe....I'll Repeat These 3 Affirmations Today:

1. _____

2. _____

3. _____

My Gratitude Journal (every day I list something new):

1. _____

2. _____

3. _____

My Daily Stats (optional):

Weight: _____   Blood Sugar: _____   Other: _____

Blood
Pressure: _____   Cholesterol: _____   Other: _____

My Daily Fitness Activity:

Activity	Duration

Daily Food Checklist & Journal

Cycle 2, Day 10 Date: _____ (Accelerate Day)	Daily Food Journal (Food Types and Quantities)
Breakfast: ☐ Protein and/or Probiotics ☐ Fruit	
Lunch: ☐ Protein and/or Probiotics ☐ Cleansing Vegetables	
Dinner: ☐ Protein ☐ Cleansing Vegetables	
Snacks: ☐ 2nd Probiotic ☐ 2nd Fruit before 2pm	
Friendly Fats (2 Servings): ☐ Olive/Flax Oil	

Daily Hydration Check	
Hot Lemon Water	☐
Plain Water	☐ ☐ ☐ ☐ ☐ ☐ ☐
Green Tea	☐ ☐ ☐

Working from the Inside Out

Cycle 2, Day 11 Date: _____

My Daily Intention: how do I want to feel today?

I Believe....I'll Repeat These 3 Affirmations Today:

1. _____

2. _____

3. _____

My Gratitude Journal (every day I list something new):

1. _____

2. _____

3. _____

My Daily Stats (optional):

Weight: _____   Blood Sugar: _____   Other: _____

Blood
Pressure: _____   Cholesterol: _____   Other: _____

My Daily Fitness Activity:

Activity	Duration

Daily Food Checklist & Journal

Cycle 2, Day 11 Date: _____ (Activate Day)	Daily Food Journal (Food Types and Quantities)
Breakfast: ☐ Protein and/or Probiotics ☐ Fruit ☐ Natural Starch	
Lunch: ☐ Protein and/or Probiotics ☐ Cleansing Vegetables ☐ Natural Starch	
Dinner: ☐ Protein ☐ Cleansing Vegetables	
Snacks: ☐ 2nd Probiotic ☐ 2nd Fruit before 2pm	
Friendly Fats (2 Servings): ☐ Olive/Flax Oil	

Daily Hydration Check	
Hot Lemon Water	☐
Plain Water	☐ ☐ ☐ ☐ ☐ ☐ ☐
Green Tea	☐ ☐ ☐

Working from the Inside Out

Cycle 2, Day 12 Date: _____

My Daily Intention: how do I want to feel today?

I Believe....I'll Repeat These 3 Affirmations Today:

1. _____

2. _____

3. _____

My Gratitude Journal (every day I list something new):

1. _____

2. _____

3. _____

My Daily Stats (optional):

Weight: _____   Blood Sugar: _____   Other: _____

Blood
Pressure: _____   Cholesterol: _____   Other: _____

My Daily Fitness Activity:

Activity	Duration

Daily Food Checklist & Journal

Cycle 2, Day 12 Date: _____ (Accelerate Day)	Daily Food Journal (Food Types and Quantities)
Breakfast: ☐ Protein and/or Probiotics ☐ Fruit	
Lunch: ☐ Protein and/or Probiotics ☐ Cleansing Vegetables	
Dinner: ☐ Protein ☐ Cleansing Vegetables	
Snacks: ☐ 2nd Probiotic ☐ 2nd Fruit before 2pm	
Friendly Fats (2 Servings): ☐ Olive/Flax Oil	

Daily Hydration Check	
Hot Lemon Water	☐
Plain Water	☐ ☐ ☐ ☐ ☐ ☐ ☐ ☐
Green Tea	☐ ☐ ☐

Working from the Inside Out

Cycle 2, Day 13 Date: _____

My Daily Intention: how do I want to feel today?

I Believe....I'll Repeat These 3 Affirmations Today:

1. _____

2. _____

3. _____

My Gratitude Journal (every day I list something new):

1. _____

2. _____

3. _____

My Daily Stats (optional):

Weight: _____   Blood Sugar: _____   Other: _____

Blood
Pressure: _____   Cholesterol: _____   Other: _____

My Daily Fitness Activity:

Activity	Duration

Daily Food Checklist & Journal

Cycle 2, Day 13 Date: _____ (Activate Day)	Daily Food Journal (Food Types and Quantities)
Breakfast: ☐ Protein and/or Probiotics ☐ Fruit ☐ Natural Starch	
Lunch: ☐ Protein and/or Probiotics ☐ Cleansing Vegetables ☐ Natural Starch	
Dinner: ☐ Protein ☐ Cleansing Vegetables	
Snacks: ☐ 2nd Probiotic ☐ 2nd Fruit before 2pm	
Friendly Fats (2 Servings): ☐ Olive/Flax Oil	

Daily Hydration Check	
Hot Lemon Water	☐
Plain Water	☐ ☐ ☐ ☐ ☐ ☐ ☐
Green Tea	☐ ☐ ☐

Working from the Inside Out

Cycle 2, Day 14 Date: _____

My Daily Intention: how do I want to feel today?

I Believe....I'll Repeat These 3 Affirmations Today:

1. _____

2. _____

3. _____

My Gratitude Journal (every day I list something new):

1. _____

2. _____

3. _____

My Daily Stats (optional):

Weight: _____   Blood Sugar: _____   Other: _____

Blood
Pressure: _____   Cholesterol: _____   Other: _____

My Daily Fitness Activity:

Activity	Duration

Daily Food Checklist & Journal

Cycle 2, Day 14 Date: _____ (Accelerate Day)	Daily Food Journal (Food Types and Quantities)
Breakfast: ☐ Protein and/or Probiotics ☐ Fruit	
Lunch: ☐ Protein and/or Probiotics ☐ Cleansing Vegetables	
Dinner: ☐ Protein ☐ Cleansing Vegetables	
Snacks: ☐ 2nd Probiotic ☐ 2nd Fruit before 2pm	
Friendly Fats (2 Servings): ☐ Olive/Flax Oil	

Daily Hydration Check	
Hot Lemon Water	☐
Plain Water	☐ ☐ ☐ ☐ ☐ ☐ ☐
Green Tea	☐ ☐ ☐

Working from the Inside Out

Cycle 2, Day 15 Date: _____

My Daily Intention: how do I want to feel today?

I Believe....I'll Repeat These 3 Affirmations Today:

1. _____

2. _____

3. _____

My Gratitude Journal (every day I list something new):

1. _____

2. _____

3. _____

My Daily Stats (optional):

Weight: _____   Blood Sugar: _____   Other: _____

Blood
Pressure: _____   Cholesterol: _____   Other: _____

My Daily Fitness Activity:

Activity	Duration

Daily Food Checklist & Journal

Cycle 2, Day 15 Date: _____ (Activate Day)	Daily Food Journal (Food Types and Quantities)
Breakfast: ☐ Protein and/or Probiotics ☐ Fruit ☐ Natural Starch	
Lunch: ☐ Protein and/or Probiotics ☐ Cleansing Vegetables ☐ Natural Starch	
Dinner: ☐ Protein ☐ Cleansing Vegetables	
Snacks: ☐ 2nd Probiotic ☐ 2nd Fruit before 2pm	
Friendly Fats (2 Servings): ☐ Olive/Flax Oil	

Daily Hydration Check	
Hot Lemon Water	☐
Plain Water	☐ ☐ ☐ ☐ ☐ ☐ ☐ ☐
Green Tea	☐ ☐ ☐

Working from the Inside Out

Cycle 2, Day 16 Date: _____

My Daily Intention: how do I want to feel today?

I Believe....I'll Repeat These 3 Affirmations Today:

1. _____

2. _____

3. _____

My Gratitude Journal (every day I list something new):

1. _____

2. _____

3. _____

My Daily Stats (optional):

Weight: _____   Blood Sugar: _____   Other: _____

Blood
Pressure: _____   Cholesterol: _____   Other: _____

My Daily Fitness Activity:

Activity	Duration

Daily Food Checklist & Journal

Cycle 2, Day 16 Date: _____ (Accelerate Day)	Daily Food Journal (Food Types and Quantities)
Breakfast: ☐ Protein and/or Probiotics ☐ Fruit	
Lunch: ☐ Protein and/or Probiotics ☐ Cleansing Vegetables	
Dinner: ☐ Protein ☐ Cleansing Vegetables	
Snacks: ☐ 2nd Probiotic ☐ 2nd Fruit before 2pm	
Friendly Fats (2 Servings): ☐ Olive/Flax Oil	

Daily Hydration Check	
Hot Lemon Water	☐
Plain Water	☐ ☐ ☐ ☐ ☐ ☐ ☐ ☐
Green Tea	☐ ☐ ☐

Working from the Inside Out

Cycle 2, Day 17 Date: _____

My Daily Intention: how do I want to feel today?

I Believe....I'll Repeat These 3 Affirmations Today:

1. _____

2. _____

3. _____

My Gratitude Journal (every day I list something new):

1. _____

2. _____

3. _____

My Daily Stats (optional):

Weight: _____   Blood Sugar: _____   Other: _____

Blood
Pressure: _____   Cholesterol: _____   Other: _____

My Daily Fitness Activity:

Activity	Duration

Daily Food Checklist & Journal

Cycle 2, Day 17 Date: _____ (Activate Day)	Daily Food Journal (Food Types and Quantities)
Breakfast: ☐ Protein and/or Probiotics ☐ Fruit ☐ Natural Starch	
Lunch: ☐ Protein and/or Probiotics ☐ Cleansing Vegetables ☐ Natural Starch	
Dinner: ☐ Protein ☐ Cleansing Vegetables	
Snacks: ☐ 2nd Probiotic ☐ 2nd Fruit before 2pm	
Friendly Fats (2 Servings): ☐ Olive/Flax Oil	

Daily Hydration Check	
Hot Lemon Water	☐
Plain Water	☐ ☐ ☐ ☐ ☐ ☐ ☐ ☐
Green Tea	☐ ☐ ☐

Ending Stats
Cycle 2, Days 9 - 17

Date: _____

Weight: _____

Inches:

Neck: _____   Midriff: _____

Chest: _____   Hips: _____

Left Arm: _____   Left Thigh: _____

My Wins

I celebrate the following wins (both big and small) from the last 9 days:

1. _____

2. _____

3. _____

Random Thoughts, Ideas & Musings (drawings allowed, too!)

Reflect & Review
Cycle 2, Days 1 – 17

	Beginning Stats	Ending Stats	Difference
Weight			
Inches:			
Neck			
Chest			
Left Arm			
Midriff			
Hips			
Left Thigh			

The 1 Thing

During the last 17 days of this cycle, I learned the following about myself...

Gratitude Journal

Cycle 3

Days 1 – 8

I maintain a healthy relationship with food and make better choices to nourish my body.

Beginning Stats

Cycle 3, Days 1 - 8

Date: _____

Weight: _____

Inches:

Neck: _____

Midriff: _____

Chest: _____

Hips: _____

Left Arm: _____

Left Thigh: _____

Mini Goals

I want to achieve the following 3 "mini goals" in the next 8 days:

1. _____

2. _____

3. _____

Random Thoughts, Ideas & Musings (drawings allowed, too!)

Working from the Inside Out

Cycle 3, Day 1 Date: _____

My Daily Intention: how do I want to feel today?

I Believe....I'll Repeat These 3 Affirmations Today:

1. _____

2. _____

3. _____

My Gratitude Journal (every day I list something new):

1. _____

2. _____

3. _____

My Daily Stats (optional):

Weight: _____   Blood Sugar: _____   Other: _____

Blood
Pressure: _____   Cholesterol: _____   Other: _____

My Daily Fitness Activity:

Activity	Duration

Daily Food Checklist & Journal

Cycle 3, Day 1 Date: _____	Daily Food Journal (Food Types and Quantities)
Breakfast: ☐ Protein and/or Probiotics ☐ Fruit ☐ Natural Starch	
Lunch: ☐ Protein and/or Probiotics ☐ Cleansing Vegetables ☐ Natural Starch	
Dinner: ☐ Protein ☐ Cleansing Vegetables	
Snacks: ☐ 2nd Probiotic or low-fat dairy ☐ 2nd Fruit before 2pm	
Friendly Fats (2 Servings): ☐ Olive/Flax Oil	

Daily Hydration Check	
Hot Lemon Water	☐
Plain Water	☐ ☐ ☐ ☐ ☐ ☐ ☐ ☐
Green Tea	☐ ☐ ☐

Working from the Inside Out

Cycle 3, Day 2 Date: _____

My Daily Intention: how do I want to feel today?

I Believe....I'll Repeat These 3 Affirmations Today:

1. _____

2. _____

3. _____

My Gratitude Journal (every day I list something new):

1. _____

2. _____

3. _____

My Daily Stats (optional):

Weight: _____   Blood Sugar: _____   Other: _____

Blood
Pressure: _____   Cholesterol: _____   Other: _____

My Daily Fitness Activity:

Activity	Duration

Daily Food Checklist & Journal

Cycle 3, Day 2 Date: _____	Daily Food Journal (Food Types and Quantities)
Breakfast: ☐ Protein and/or Probiotics ☐ Fruit ☐ Natural Starch	
Lunch: ☐ Protein and/or Probiotics ☐ Cleansing Vegetables ☐ Natural Starch	
Dinner: ☐ Protein ☐ Cleansing Vegetables	
Snacks: ☐ 2nd Probiotic or low-fat dairy ☐ 2nd Fruit before 2pm	
Friendly Fats (2 Servings): ☐ Olive/Flax Oil	

Daily Hydration Check	
Hot Lemon Water	☐
Plain Water	☐ ☐ ☐ ☐ ☐ ☐ ☐
Green Tea	☐ ☐ ☐

Working from the Inside Out

Cycle 3, Day 3 Date: _____

My Daily Intention: how do I want to feel today?

I Believe....I'll Repeat These 3 Affirmations Today:

1. _____

2. _____

3. _____

My Gratitude Journal (every day I list something new):

1. _____

2. _____

3. _____

My Daily Stats (optional):

Weight: _____   Blood Sugar: _____   Other: _____

Blood
Pressure: _____   Cholesterol: _____   Other: _____

My Daily Fitness Activity:

Activity	Duration

Daily Food Checklist & Journal

Cycle 3, Day 3 Date: _____	Daily Food Journal (Food Types and Quantities)
Breakfast: ☐ Protein and/or Probiotics ☐ Fruit ☐ Natural Starch	
Lunch: ☐ Protein and/or Probiotics ☐ Cleansing Vegetables ☐ Natural Starch	
Dinner: ☐ Protein ☐ Cleansing Vegetables	
Snacks: ☐ 2nd Probiotic or low-fat dairy ☐ 2nd Fruit before 2pm	
Friendly Fats (2 Servings): ☐ Olive/Flax Oil	

Daily Hydration Check	
Hot Lemon Water	☐
Plain Water	☐ ☐ ☐ ☐ ☐ ☐ ☐ ☐
Green Tea	☐ ☐ ☐

Working from the Inside Out

Cycle 3, Day 4 Date: _____

My Daily Intention: how do I want to feel today?

I Believe....I'll Repeat These 3 Affirmations Today:

1. _____

2. _____

3. _____

My Gratitude Journal (every day I list something new):

1. _____

2. _____

3. _____

My Daily Stats (optional):

Weight: _____   Blood Sugar: _____   Other: _____

Blood
Pressure: _____   Cholesterol: _____   Other: _____

My Daily Fitness Activity:

Activity	Duration

Daily Food Checklist & Journal

Cycle 3, Day 4 Date: _____	Daily Food Journal (Food Types and Quantities)
Breakfast: ☐ Protein and/or Probiotics ☐ Fruit ☐ Natural Starch	
Lunch: ☐ Protein and/or Probiotics ☐ Cleansing Vegetables ☐ Natural Starch	
Dinner: ☐ Protein ☐ Cleansing Vegetables	
Snacks: ☐ 2nd Probiotic or low-fat dairy ☐ 2nd Fruit before 2pm	
Friendly Fats (2 Servings): ☐ Olive/Flax Oil	

Daily Hydration Check	
Hot Lemon Water	☐
Plain Water	☐ ☐ ☐ ☐ ☐ ☐ ☐ ☐
Green Tea	☐ ☐ ☐

Working from the Inside Out

Cycle 3, Day 5 Date: _____

My Daily Intention: how do I want to feel today?

I Believe....I'll Repeat These 3 Affirmations Today:

1. _____

2. _____

3. _____

My Gratitude Journal (every day I list something new):

1. _____

2. _____

3. _____

My Daily Stats (optional):

Weight: _____   Blood Sugar: _____   Other: _____

Blood
Pressure: _____   Cholesterol: _____   Other: _____

My Daily Fitness Activity:

Activity	Duration

Daily Food Checklist & Journal

Cycle 3, Day 5 Date: _____	Daily Food Journal (Food Types and Quantities)
Breakfast: ☐ Protein and/or Probiotics ☐ Fruit ☐ Natural Starch	
Lunch: ☐ Protein and/or Probiotics ☐ Cleansing Vegetables ☐ Natural Starch	
Dinner: ☐ Protein ☐ Cleansing Vegetables	
Snacks: ☐ 2nd Probiotic or low-fat dairy ☐ 2nd Fruit before 2pm	
Friendly Fats (2 Servings): ☐ Olive/Flax Oil	

Daily Hydration Check	
Hot Lemon Water	☐
Plain Water	☐ ☐ ☐ ☐ ☐ ☐ ☐ ☐
Green Tea	☐ ☐ ☐

Working from the Inside Out

Cycle 3, Day 6 Date: _____

My Daily Intention: how do I want to feel today?

I Believe....I'll Repeat These 3 Affirmations Today:

1. _____

2. _____

3. _____

My Gratitude Journal (every day I list something new):

1. _____

2. _____

3. _____

My Daily Stats (optional):

Weight: _____   Blood Sugar: _____   Other: _____

Blood
Pressure: _____   Cholesterol: _____   Other: _____

My Daily Fitness Activity:

Activity	Duration

Daily Food Checklist & Journal

Cycle 3, Day 6 Date: _____	Daily Food Journal (Food Types and Quantities)
Breakfast: ☐ Protein and/or Probiotics ☐ Fruit ☐ Natural Starch	
Lunch: ☐ Protein and/or Probiotics ☐ Cleansing Vegetables ☐ Natural Starch	
Dinner: ☐ Protein ☐ Cleansing Vegetables	
Snacks: ☐ 2nd Probiotic or low-fat dairy ☐ 2nd Fruit before 2pm	
Friendly Fats (2 Servings): ☐ Olive/Flax Oil	

Daily Hydration Check	
Hot Lemon Water	☐
Plain Water	☐ ☐ ☐ ☐ ☐ ☐ ☐ ☐
Green Tea	☐ ☐ ☐

Working from the Inside Out

Cycle 3, Day 7 Date: _____

My Daily Intention: how do I want to feel today?

I Believe....I'll Repeat These 3 Affirmations Today:

1. _____

2. _____

3. _____

My Gratitude Journal (every day I list something new):

1. _____

2. _____

3. _____

My Daily Stats (optional):

Weight: _____   Blood Sugar: _____   Other: _____

Blood
Pressure: _____   Cholesterol: _____   Other: _____

My Daily Fitness Activity:

Activity	Duration

Daily Food Checklist & Journal

Cycle 3, Day 7 Date: _____	Daily Food Journal (Food Types and Quantities)
Breakfast: ☐ Protein and/or Probiotics ☐ Fruit ☐ Natural Starch	
Lunch: ☐ Protein and/or Probiotics ☐ Cleansing Vegetables ☐ Natural Starch	
Dinner: ☐ Protein ☐ Cleansing Vegetables	
Snacks: ☐ 2nd Probiotic or low-fat dairy ☐ 2nd Fruit before 2pm	
Friendly Fats (2 Servings): ☐ Olive/Flax Oil	

Daily Hydration Check	
Hot Lemon Water	☐
Plain Water	☐ ☐ ☐ ☐ ☐ ☐ ☐ ☐
Green Tea	☐ ☐ ☐

Working from the Inside Out

Cycle 3, Day 8 Date: _____

My Daily Intention: how do I want to feel today?

I Believe....I'll Repeat These 3 Affirmations Today:

1. _____

2. _____

3. _____

My Gratitude Journal (every day I list something new):

1. _____

2. _____

3. _____

My Daily Stats (optional):

Weight: _____ Blood Sugar: _____ Other: _____

Blood
Pressure: _____ Cholesterol: _____ Other: _____

My Daily Fitness Activity:

Activity	Duration

Daily Food Checklist & Journal

Cycle 3, Day 8 Date: _____	Daily Food Journal (Food Types and Quantities)
Breakfast: ☐ Protein and/or Probiotics ☐ Fruit ☐ Natural Starch	
Lunch: ☐ Protein and/or Probiotics ☐ Cleansing Vegetables ☐ Natural Starch	
Dinner: ☐ Protein ☐ Cleansing Vegetables	
Snacks: ☐ 2nd Probiotic or low-fat dairy ☐ 2nd Fruit before 2pm	
Friendly Fats (2 Servings): ☐ Olive/Flax Oil	

Daily Hydration Check	
Hot Lemon Water	☐
Plain Water	☐ ☐ ☐ ☐ ☐ ☐ ☐ ☐
Green Tea	☐ ☐ ☐

Ending Stats
Cycle 3, Days 1 - 8

Date: _____

Weight: _____

Inches:

Neck: _____   Midriff: _____

Chest: _____   Hips: _____

Left Arm: _____   Left Thigh: _____

My Wins

I celebrate the following wins (both big and small) from the last 8 days:

1. _____

2. _____

3. _____

Random Thoughts, Ideas & Musings (drawings allowed, too!)

Cycle 3

Days 9 – 17

I am in awe of the progress I've made in such a short amount of time. I acknowledge small, actionable steps daily will allow me to achieve extraordinary results.

Beginning Stats

Cycle 3, Days 9 - 17

Date: _____

Weight: _____

Inches:

Neck: _____   Midriff: _____

Chest: _____   Hips: _____

Left Arm: _____   Left Thigh: _____

Mini Goals

I want to achieve the following 3 "mini goals" in the next 9 days:

1. _____

2. _____

3. _____

Random Thoughts, Ideas & Musings (drawings allowed, too!)

Working from the Inside Out

Cycle 3, Day 9 Date: _____

My Daily Intention: how do I want to feel today?

I Believe....I'll Repeat These 3 Affirmations Today:

1. _____

2. _____

3. _____

My Gratitude Journal (every day I list something new):

1. _____

2. _____

3. _____

My Daily Stats (optional):

Weight: _____   Blood Sugar: _____   Other: _____

Blood
Pressure: _____   Cholesterol: _____   Other: _____

My Daily Fitness Activity:

Activity	Duration

Daily Food Checklist & Journal

Cycle 3, Day 9 Date: _____	Daily Food Journal (Food Types and Quantities)
Breakfast: ☐ Protein and/or Probiotics ☐ Fruit ☐ Natural Starch	
Lunch: ☐ Protein and/or Probiotics ☐ Cleansing Vegetables ☐ Natural Starch	
Dinner: ☐ Protein ☐ Cleansing Vegetables	
Snacks: ☐ 2nd Probiotic or low-fat dairy ☐ 2nd Fruit before 2pm	
Friendly Fats (2 Servings): ☐ Olive/Flax Oil	

Daily Hydration Check	
Hot Lemon Water	☐
Plain Water	☐ ☐ ☐ ☐ ☐ ☐ ☐ ☐
Green Tea	☐ ☐ ☐

Working from the Inside Out

Cycle 3, Day 10 Date: _____

My Daily Intention: how do I want to feel today?

I Believe....I'll Repeat These 3 Affirmations Today:

1. _____

2. _____

3. _____

My Gratitude Journal (every day I list something new):

1. _____

2. _____

3. _____

My Daily Stats (optional):

Weight: _____   Blood Sugar: _____   Other: _____

Blood
Pressure: _____   Cholesterol: _____   Other: _____

My Daily Fitness Activity:

Activity	Duration

Daily Food Checklist & Journal

Cycle 3, Day 10 Date: _____	Daily Food Journal (Food Types and Quantities)
Breakfast: ☐ Protein and/or Probiotics ☐ Fruit ☐ Natural Starch	
Lunch: ☐ Protein and/or Probiotics ☐ Cleansing Vegetables ☐ Natural Starch	
Dinner: ☐ Protein ☐ Cleansing Vegetables	
Snacks: ☐ 2nd Probiotic or low-fat dairy ☐ 2nd Fruit before 2pm	
Friendly Fats (2 Servings): ☐ Olive/Flax Oil	

Daily Hydration Check	
Hot Lemon Water	☐
Plain Water	☐ ☐ ☐ ☐ ☐ ☐ ☐ ☐
Green Tea	☐ ☐ ☐

Working from the Inside Out

Cycle 3, Day 11 Date: _____

My Daily Intention: how do I want to feel today?

I Believe....I'll Repeat These 3 Affirmations Today:

1. _____

2. _____

3. _____

My Gratitude Journal (every day I list something new):

1. _____

2. _____

3. _____

My Daily Stats (optional):

Weight: _____   Blood Sugar: _____   Other: _____

Blood
Pressure: _____   Cholesterol: _____   Other: _____

My Daily Fitness Activity:

Activity	Duration

Daily Food Checklist & Journal

Cycle 3, Day 11 Date: _____	Daily Food Journal (Food Types and Quantities)
Breakfast: ☐ Protein and/or Probiotics ☐ Fruit ☐ Natural Starch	
Lunch: ☐ Protein and/or Probiotics ☐ Cleansing Vegetables ☐ Natural Starch	
Dinner: ☐ Protein ☐ Cleansing Vegetables	
Snacks: ☐ 2nd Probiotic or low-fat dairy ☐ 2nd Fruit before 2pm	
Friendly Fats (2 Servings): ☐ Olive/Flax Oil	

Daily Hydration Check	
Hot Lemon Water	☐
Plain Water	☐ ☐ ☐ ☐ ☐ ☐ ☐
Green Tea	☐ ☐ ☐

Working from the Inside Out

Cycle 3, Day 12 Date: _____

My Daily Intention: how do I want to feel today?

I Believe....I'll Repeat These 3 Affirmations Today:

1. _____

2. _____

3. _____

My Gratitude Journal (every day I list something new):

1. _____

2. _____

3. _____

My Daily Stats (optional):

Weight: _____   Blood Sugar: _____   Other: _____

Blood
Pressure: _____   Cholesterol: _____   Other: _____

My Daily Fitness Activity:

Activity	Duration

Daily Food Checklist & Journal

Cycle 3, Day 12 Date: _____	Daily Food Journal (Food Types and Quantities)
Breakfast: ☐ Protein and/or Probiotics ☐ Fruit ☐ Natural Starch	
Lunch: ☐ Protein and/or Probiotics ☐ Cleansing Vegetables ☐ Natural Starch	
Dinner: ☐ Protein ☐ Cleansing Vegetables	
Snacks: ☐ 2nd Probiotic or low-fat dairy ☐ 2nd Fruit before 2pm	
Friendly Fats (2 Servings): ☐ Olive/Flax Oil	

Daily Hydration Check	
Hot Lemon Water	☐
Plain Water	☐ ☐ ☐ ☐ ☐ ☐ ☐ ☐
Green Tea	☐ ☐ ☐

Working from the Inside Out

Cycle 3, Day 13 Date: _____

My Daily Intention: how do I want to feel today?

I Believe....I'll Repeat These 3 Affirmations Today:

1. _____

2. _____

3. _____

My Gratitude Journal (every day I list something new):

1. _____

2. _____

3. _____

My Daily Stats (optional):

Weight: _____   Blood Sugar: _____   Other: _____

Blood
Pressure: _____   Cholesterol: _____   Other: _____

My Daily Fitness Activity:

Activity	Duration

Daily Food Checklist & Journal

Cycle 3, Day 13 Date: _____	Daily Food Journal (Food Types and Quantities)
Breakfast: ☐ Protein and/or Probiotics ☐ Fruit ☐ Natural Starch	
Lunch: ☐ Protein and/or Probiotics ☐ Cleansing Vegetables ☐ Natural Starch	
Dinner: ☐ Protein ☐ Cleansing Vegetables	
Snacks: ☐ 2nd Probiotic or low-fat dairy ☐ 2nd Fruit before 2pm	
Friendly Fats (2 Servings): ☐ Olive/Flax Oil	

Daily Hydration Check	
Hot Lemon Water	☐
Plain Water	☐ ☐ ☐ ☐ ☐ ☐ ☐
Green Tea	☐ ☐ ☐

Working from the Inside Out

Cycle 3, Day 14 Date: _____

My Daily Intention: how do I want to feel today?

I Believe....I'll Repeat These 3 Affirmations Today:

1. _____

2. _____

3. _____

My Gratitude Journal (every day I list something new):

1. _____

2. _____

3. _____

My Daily Stats (optional):

Weight: _____   Blood Sugar: _____   Other: _____

Blood
Pressure: _____   Cholesterol: _____   Other: _____

My Daily Fitness Activity:

Activity	Duration

Daily Food Checklist & Journal

Cycle 3, Day 14 Date: _____	Daily Food Journal (Food Types and Quantities)
Breakfast: ☐ Protein and/or Probiotics ☐ Fruit ☐ Natural Starch	
Lunch: ☐ Protein and/or Probiotics ☐ Cleansing Vegetables ☐ Natural Starch	
Dinner: ☐ Protein ☐ Cleansing Vegetables	
Snacks: ☐ 2nd Probiotic or low-fat dairy ☐ 2nd Fruit before 2pm	
Friendly Fats (2 Servings): ☐ Olive/Flax Oil	

Daily Hydration Check	
Hot Lemon Water	☐
Plain Water	☐ ☐ ☐ ☐ ☐ ☐ ☐ ☐
Green Tea	☐ ☐ ☐

Working from the Inside Out

Cycle 3, Day 15 Date: _____

My Daily Intention: how do I want to feel today?

I Believe....I'll Repeat These 3 Affirmations Today:

1. _____

2. _____

3. _____

My Gratitude Journal (every day I list something new):

1. _____

2. _____

3. _____

My Daily Stats (optional):

Weight: _____   Blood Sugar: _____   Other: _____

Blood
Pressure: _____   Cholesterol: _____   Other: _____

My Daily Fitness Activity:

Activity	Duration

Daily Food Checklist & Journal

Cycle 3, Day 15 Date: _____	Daily Food Journal (Food Types and Quantities)
Breakfast: ☐ Protein and/or Probiotics ☐ Fruit ☐ Natural Starch	
Lunch: ☐ Protein and/or Probiotics ☐ Cleansing Vegetables ☐ Natural Starch	
Dinner: ☐ Protein ☐ Cleansing Vegetables	
Snacks: ☐ 2nd Probiotic or low-fat dairy ☐ 2nd Fruit before 2pm	
Friendly Fats (2 Servings): ☐ Olive/Flax Oil	

Daily Hydration Check	
Hot Lemon Water	☐
Plain Water	☐ ☐ ☐ ☐ ☐ ☐ ☐
Green Tea	☐ ☐ ☐

Working from the Inside Out

Cycle 3, Day 16 Date: _____

My Daily Intention: how do I want to feel today?

I Believe....I'll Repeat These 3 Affirmations Today:

1. _____

2. _____

3. _____

My Gratitude Journal (every day I list something new):

1. _____

2. _____

3. _____

My Daily Stats (optional):

Weight: _____   Blood Sugar: _____   Other: _____

Blood
Pressure: _____   Cholesterol: _____   Other: _____

My Daily Fitness Activity:

Activity	Duration

Daily Food Checklist & Journal

Cycle 3, Day 16 Date: _____	Daily Food Journal (Food Types and Quantities)
Breakfast: ☐ Protein and/or Probiotics ☐ Fruit ☐ Natural Starch	
Lunch: ☐ Protein and/or Probiotics ☐ Cleansing Vegetables ☐ Natural Starch	
Dinner: ☐ Protein ☐ Cleansing Vegetables	
Snacks: ☐ 2nd Probiotic or low-fat dairy ☐ 2nd Fruit before 2pm	
Friendly Fats (2 Servings): ☐ Olive/Flax Oil	

Daily Hydration Check	
Hot Lemon Water	☐
Plain Water	☐ ☐ ☐ ☐ ☐ ☐ ☐ ☐
Green Tea	☐ ☐ ☐

Working from the Inside Out

Cycle 3, Day 17 Date: _____

My Daily Intention: how do I want to feel today?

I Believe....I'll Repeat These 3 Affirmations Today:

1. _____

2. _____

3. _____

My Gratitude Journal (every day I list something new):

1. _____

2. _____

3. _____

My Daily Stats (optional):

Weight: _____   Blood Sugar: _____   Other: _____

Blood
Pressure: _____   Cholesterol: _____   Other: _____

My Daily Fitness Activity:

Activity	Duration

Daily Food Checklist & Journal

Cycle 3, Day 17 Date: _____	Daily Food Journal (Food Types and Quantities)
Breakfast: ☐ Protein and/or Probiotics ☐ Fruit ☐ Natural Starch	
Lunch: ☐ Protein and/or Probiotics ☐ Cleansing Vegetables ☐ Natural Starch	
Dinner: ☐ Protein ☐ Cleansing Vegetables	
Snacks: ☐ 2nd Probiotic or low-fat dairy ☐ 2nd Fruit before 2pm	
Friendly Fats (2 Servings): ☐ Olive/Flax Oil	

Daily Hydration Check	
Hot Lemon Water	☐
Plain Water	☐ ☐ ☐ ☐ ☐ ☐ ☐
Green Tea	☐ ☐ ☐

Ending Stats
Cycle 3, Days 9 - 17

Date: _____

Weight: _____

Inches:

Neck: _____   Midriff: _____

Chest: _____   Hips: _____

Left Arm: _____   Left Thigh: _____

My Wins

I celebrate the following wins (both big and small) from the last 9 days:

1. _____

2. _____

3. _____

Random Thoughts, Ideas & Musings (drawings allowed, too!)

Reflect & Review
Cycle 3, Days 1 – 17

	Beginning Stats	Ending Stats	Difference
Weight			
Inches:			
Neck			
Chest			
Left Arm			
Midriff			
Hips			
Left Thigh			

The 1 Thing

During the last 17 days of this cycle, I learned the following about myself...

Gratitude Journal

This might be the end of the journal, but it's really only the beginning. Enjoy the ride!

ABOUT THE AUTHOR

Torey Lynn specializes in digital publishing with an emphasis on helping busy women save time, stay motivated and see results with the 17 Day Diet.

Torey's mission is to empower every woman to know her self worth and to believe she can accomplish anything in life.

As founder and publisher of 17 Day Lifestyle Magazine and 17ddblog.com, Torey's main focus is simplifying and organizing the 17 Day Diet by providing meal plans and easy-to-make recipes with her signature meal plan, Simple N' Lean 17, and through her weekly meal planning service, Simply17. Say hello to Torey over at 17ddblog.com.

Made in the USA
Coppell, TX
10 April 2021